THE TRAINING GUIDE I WISH I HAD

HN RANDY L. HUGHES II

RANDY HUGHES

TABLE OF CONTENTS

ABOUT ME 7

WHAT YOU SHOULD KNOW 8

50 TO PASS, 70 TO ELEVATE 9

TRAINING 11
    THE SWIM: 11
    PUSH, SIT, PULL 14
    THE PUSH-UP: 14
    THE SIT-UP: 15
    THE PULL-UP: 15
    THE RUN 16
    THE PST CLOSING THOUGHTS 18

WRITE IT DOWN 19

THINGS I WISH I DID BEFORE SHIPPING OFF THE MILITARY 20
    OCEAN SWIMMING 21
    EGG BEATER 21
    SHAVE THE CALLUS 22

THINGS LEARNED GOING THROUGH TRAINING 23
    STRIP YOUR BOOTS 23
    GEAR ISSUE 25
    PETROLEUM JELLY 26
    SAVE YOUR PISS 26
    SUPER GLUE TREATMENT 27
    FOOD 28
    HYDRATE 31
    MAKE THEM LAUGH 31
    BE EXCITED TO BE THERE 34
    I SHOULD HAVE SAID NO! 36

PEOPLE ARE GOING TO QUIT 38

DROPPED FROM TRAINING. NOW WHAT? 40

BUD/S BOX 41

STOLEN GEAR 44

LAST WORD 45

OFFICIAL PST LOG **46**

MOCK PST **48**

MEAL TRACKER **50**

THE TRAINIG GUIDE I WISH I HAD

ABOUT ME

My name is Randy Hughes. I am a 6-year Navy veteran and once was an S.W.C.C. candidate. I left my hometown of Las Vegas, Nevada, in October 2015 with the golden ticket, S.W.C.C. candidate contract. After completing Bootcamp, I spent 8 additional weeks in Great Mistakes at the preparatory school before moving to San Diego, California. While in prep school, I would receive the number 90. This was my class number. The Bud/s class for Seal candidates was 318. After completing the 8-week prep course, we left for the real deal, the compound. It was there that my journey would end. I was performance dropped due to evolution failures. Though I didn't make it through training and become an operator, I have learned many things. Some of these things I wish I knew I was going through the aspiring journey.

WHAT YOU SHOULD KNOW

So, you want to be an operator? That's nice. According to the statistics, you won't make it. This training is no joke. It's hard, it's taxing. The training will tax you mentally and physically. It's abusive. You won't know which body parts ache and which ones don't. You will be told over and over to QUIT. DO NOT QUIT! One more time for the guys in the back. <u>DO NOT FUCKING QUIT!!!</u>

Seal and S.W.C.C. training is part of what the Navy called "Warrior Programs." This is somewhat of a scouting program of the Navy. They don't tell you it is one of the Navy's best recruitment tools. Check this out: a movie about Navy Seals is made. Many young men, roughly high school/college, see this movie and are hyped. They want to be like the bad MFers they saw on the silver screen. They walk into the recruiter's office and tell the Petty Officer behind the desk they are feeling froggy. Some months later, many find their asses in training, and they do exactly what I told you never to do, quit. What happens now? You reclassified to another job in the World's Greatest Navy. Out of a class of around 300 candidates, only maybe 6 graduate on their quest to become operators. The Navy just supplied the fleet with 294 disgruntled sailors who had the shit kicked out of them and their dreams crushed. This was the only time I cried in the Navy, March 15, 2016.

50 TO PASS, 70 TO ELEVATE

When you pass the A.S.V.A.B. testing and go through the military processing, you will have x number of months to receive a candidate contract for SEAL, S.W.C.C., E.O.D., DIVER, or A.I.R. The recruiter will send you to a Mentor. He will be either on active duty or a retired seal. He will proctor your tests. I had one who would come to my hometown every other week for three days. We would use the public lap pool. He would lead Physical Training (P.T.) on Wednesday and Thursday. Friday was test day. He would show up at 0500. Everyone else was to be there before that time. We would have to check with him to have our names put on the roster. This activity was usually done in the lean and rest. After doing this, we would warm up and stretch. The mentor would sit in the car and blare Hotel California and rev the engine during the winter months.

At 0530, The lifeguards would unlock the gate and let us in. The test began with a 500-yard swim followed by push-ups, sit-ups, pull-ups, and a 1.5-mile run. Competing for contracts is highly competitive and gets more so as the years go by. You want the golden ticket; you will earn it. The Navy issues a certain of contracts per year. You are competing against a bunch of guys just like you. Your competition is those in your group and those around the country. So, you must put up competitive scores. 9:30-70-70-15-10:30, this was ingrained in my head. Sub 9:30 swim, 70 push-ups, 70 sit-ups, 15 pull-ups, and sub 10:30 1.5 mile run. Our mentor would say 50 to pass 70 to elevate. 50 was the passing score for push-ups and sit-ups, but 70 for each evolution needed to be obtained to be competitive.

Once you submit good scores, you will wait to hear from your recruiter on whether you got selected by the board. If selected, you will sign a new contract for the respective pipeline. With a new training contract signed, you wait to ship out. The new contract will replace the job you picked before being selected. If you were not selected, you will keep trying until you ship out to Bootcamp. Don't think that once you get your new contract, you can get relaxed on training. At some point, before you ship off to boot camp, you will be required to perform another PST. Failure of the test can result in the loss of contract. During the final PST, I was required to complete the 500-yard swim WITHOUT a dive mask. Once you secure the contract, I recommend you practice swimming without the mask.

TRAINING

I advise you to start training before entering the recruiter's office. Like everyone else, I wanted to be a Seal. My swim time was great, but my run time wasn't enough to get the seal candidate contract. So, when I was offered an S.W.C.C. Candidate Contract, I took it. 2 years is the amount of time I gave myself to train to attempt this unique challenge.

The Swim:

I had to learn the combat sidestroke. This stroke is used during the test, which you will later use in training. I remember watching a video of this navy seal teaching how to do the Combat Side Stroke. I then found a public lap pool. I would change into swim attire and sit poolside, where I would watch the video again. I would get in the pool and attempt the stroke. I went back to the video again and again. Eventually, I could swim from one side to the other, 25 yards. Once I was competent, I would attempt one lap, down and back. After getting the technique and muscle memory down, I worked on stamina. I worked on doing lap after lap without stopping, wrapping it up, and getting the time down.

It would take me around 15 minutes to complete the 500-yard swim. That is nowhere near the time I would need. Not even close. I needed to look at my swim and figure out how to tune it to reduce time. One way my swim became more efficient was found in the beginning, The push off and glide. In the last few seconds, before the swim started, everyone would grab the wall and place their feet on the underwater portion of the wall. Everyone would submerge underwater after being given the command to begin the swim. Launch the body like a missile under the water's surface with a strong push from the legs. After the push-off, allow the body to glide. The glide should carry the body about a third to halfway across the length of a 25-yard pool—the push-off alone clips off a few seconds. If done every time you come to the wall, swim time is reduced dramatically. When I approached the wall, I would grab it and pull myself into it. I would set my feet just like I had done at the beginning. As I did this, I would inhale big, submerge myself, and push off again. Remember, you can not do flips at the wall.

Coupling with the glide after the push-off was the pull-out. This is done by stretching the arms above the head and pulling each arm down toward the sides of the body. This evolution mimics a bird flapping its wings or performing jumping jacks without using the legs. At the time, we were allowed to do a maximum of 2 pull-outs per push-off. Putting these steps together and performing them every time I meet the wall drastically lowered my swim time. This also helps preserve my energy for the evolutions following the swim.

During pool work, there were things that I did that helped enormously. First, I would begin the workout with a timed 500-yard swim. This is an excellent warm-up. The next thing I would do is a trick my father taught me: quarters. When I swam, I wouldn't keep my thumb "glued" to my index finger. When my hand was open, it created drag and slowed my swim. I would put a quarter between my thumb and index finger to train myself to hold my hand closed. I would swim like this. After a while, the muscle memory to keep my hands closed and the quarters weren't needed any longer.

Another thing that helped me swim was filming my swim or having someone watch me swim. Filming swims is good for identifying issues that add time instead of subtracting. Swerving in the lane, drifting from side to side during the swim, adds distance and time to each lap. By filming or having someone watching, I get feedback and knowledge of issues to pay more attention to certain areas. The camera doesn't lie. Maybe I'm only pushing the wall half the time. Due to video evidence, that fact will hit me every time I meet the wall.

Pro tip: Get yourself a pair of the Jammers; they are skin swim trunks that help you be more streamlined by reducing drag. You can't wear the banana hammock or man bikini, but the jammers are authorized. I used to call them my "Sexy Pants".

Push, Sit, Pull

The next evolution starts 10 minutes after the last guy leaves the pool. You will often hear this phrase: IT PAYS TO BE A WINNER! If I complete the swim sooner than others, I will have more time to rest while changing out of my sexy pants. This evolution starts with push-ups, followed by sit-ups, and finishes with pull-ups. This is a timed evolution consisting of 2 minutes of push-ups and 2 minutes of sit-ups. There is a two-minute rest period after the push-ups and the sit-ups. Practicing in front of a mirror or recording a video of the exercise is a good idea.
After completing the "push, sit, pull" there is a 10-minute rest period before the last evolution, the run.

The Push-up:

The push-up is done with the hand placed on the deck shoulder-width apart. The back is flat, and the eyes are up. Feet are together, and ass is not in the air. Upon being given the command to begin, lower the upper body toward the ground until the elbow breaks a 90-degree angle. Once achieved, raise the body upwards and lockout elbows. At no time does either hand or foot break contact with the deck. Perform the exercise until 2 minutes have expired or until failure. Only perfect push-ups count and remember 50 push-ups to pass the test, but 70+ is competitive.

The Sit-up:

This is done by lying flat on the back with feet flat on the deck 6 inches from the buttocks. Arms crossed and hands rested flat on the opposing shoulder. Raise the upper body to a sitting position until elbows contact the area between the knee and 3 inches above the knee. Once achieved, lower the body to the start position. Repeat the movement until the 2 minutes have expired or until failure. Again, 50 sit-ups are required to pass the test, but 70+ is necessary to be competitive.

The Pull-up:

The pull-up is done by mounting the bar. You are gripping with arms about shoulder-width apart. Pull the body upward towards the bar from a dead hang until the chin comes over the bar; once you have your chin past the bar, lower your body back down to the starting position. Kipping is not allowed. Repeat the movement until failure and dismount of the bar.

When working on pull-ups, I would do them pyramid-style. Mount the bar, do 1 pull-up, dismount. Mount the bar, do 2 pull-ups, dismount. Mount the bar, do 3 pull-ups, dismount. Repeat this process by doing one more pull-up than the prior set until you have done a set of 10 pull-ups. Once I had done the 10 pull-up set, I went backward. 10 then 9,8…1. If doing this solo, I would wait about 7-10 sec between each set. If I were working out with someone else, as soon as (I mean without hesitation) they dismounted the bar, I'd be back on the bar cranking out the next set.

The Run

The run is 1.5 miles in length. To lower my run time, I would run several miles a day. I would go to a giant field in the local park and run the perimeter for an hour and a half. I did this several times a week. After running, I would run the bleacher steps. Running bleachers trained me to keep my knees high when I ran, helping to cover more distance with each stride. A good idea would be to run in a place that has hills along the way. These running tips will help with building stamina.

Running in boots is something you should consider doing. While at boot camp and prep, you will run in tennis shoes. I always preferred bare minimum shoes—very lightweight and one that I could bend in half. I also found that indoor soccer shoes had a low profile. When you move on in training, it's all boots. I would run in boots a few times weekly, slowly building distance. Start with roughly a mile. You don't want to do too much too quickly. That's a recipe for screwing yourself. The focus wasn't on running a marathon in boots and pants but on getting used to running with boots and pants.

The PST Closing Thoughts

Numerous websites have the minimum scores needed to pass the test. Though you will pass the test, you will not get selected. Like I said before, the market for a contract is very competitive. You must break out. To prepare for PSTs, I have conducted mock PSTs on my own. I would run through the entire PST from start to finish. I would do a swim followed by a 10-minute rest. When 10 minutes expire, start the push-ups for 2 minutes, then a 2-minute rest. When the 2 minutes pass, begin 2 minutes of sit-ups followed by another 2-minute rest. After the 2-minute rest, mount the bar and knock out the pull-ups. Rest for 10 minutes. Lastly, as soon as the 10 minutes expire, I begin running. This PST should take you less than an hour from start to finish. One of three issues exists if it takes you longer than 44 minutes. One, you ignored the rest periods. Two, you're playing around. Third, you are too slow. The issue of being too slow can be fixed by looking at times for the swim and the run and figuring out how to reduce times. After I ran through the whole PST, I would do it again. Back-to-back PSTs help me build endurance.

I'm not going to explain how to do the Combat Side Stroke. It would be better to watch a video on the internet. There was only one video out when I was learning, and now there are many videos. Maybe one day I will make a video on it. I advise watching a few of them and hitting the pool, preferably one with a depth of 3 feet. This way, you can stand when things go wrong, recoup yourself, and begin again. Once comfortable, move to a deep area.

Write It Down

If you didn't write it down, it never happened. This phrase has stuck with me my whole Navy career. In the military, there is a logbook for just about everything. When going on the post, coming off the post, incidents, events, etc. When taking out weapons, equipment, tools, etc., log books tell a story of when and what has occurred.

I logged it every time I worked out, swam, or did calisthenics. Each time I did a formal PST, I asked for the results and logged them in my notebook. Same with every mock PST, while I'm resting, I'm logging. Get the hint? Log it. A log is an honest record. If I do poorly on the PST, I can look back and see what I did and figure out why I did poorly. This logbook holds me accountable when it comes to test time. I could have done poorly solely because it was just a bad day. This is a rare case, though.

To keep the record honest, correctly writing the count or time, whether a good number or terrible, is significant. You don't do yourself any favors by reporting a lower time than you put up. Nor when you say a higher calisthenics count. This includes counting other than perfect push-ups, sit-ups, or pull-ups. I write everything down, and everything is timed. My entries go into the logbook right after I complete the evolution. Don't let several hours pass, and then realize you didn't log your scores. Now you're trying to remember the numbers. Those numbers can't be trusted.

THINGS I WISH I DID BEFORE SHIPPING OFF THE MILITARY

WARNING: The things that I discuss are things I wish I had done. These are personal views based on what I did during training. There are things I wish I had practiced before leaving for the military. To be clear, you will never be entirely ready for the hell you will endure. People die at BUDS training. Some of this material is considered dangerous and not condoned. I am not responsible for the actions of others. This is for information purposes only. You should seek professional instruction and guidance before and during training.

Ocean Swimming

One thing that I wish I had done is ocean swimming. There are groups of people who ocean swim with wetsuits and fins. Being a part of one of these groups would have helped me a lot with swimming when it came to training. In training and during certain operations, swims are conducted with fins. Getting used to wearing and using fins before training helps a lot. I lived in Las Vegas, Nevada. There is no ocean in Las Vegas. I would practice in the pool with fins. This only does so much for you. In the swimming pool, there are no waves, no current. The water is calm compared to the open water. This also would have helped with guiding during the swim. Participating in other activities, such as diving, would be a fun and great way to get fin time and open water experience. Ocean swimming before the military would have helped me greatly.

Egg Beater

Another thing I wish I had practiced was treading water. Before leaving for the Navy, I didn't know the "egg beater" or how to do it. We would have to tread water while holding a diving brick in training. I managed to keep the brick above water while scissor kicking. Though this was effective, I still wish I was proficient at the "egg beater". Joining a water polo team could help tremendously. We had one time when we played water polo during training. When you are concentrating on the game while using what you learned to tread water, you develop more profound muscle memory.

Shave the Callus

Performing gripping evolutions such as pull-ups, a callus will develop on the upper part of the palm. I didn't know how to manage my hands or knew I needed to. It wasn't till after I was dropped from the training. There was a master chief who would hold a workout circuit before work. He told me to take an old facial razor and make several passes over the calluses. This simple trick is one that I wish I had known. This would have saved hands during training. I had torn the calluses out of both of my hands, four deep wounds on each hand.

The salt-laced sand would fill the wounds whenever we got dropped on the beach. The burning sensation was painful. The same pain happened when we were told to "hit the surf". The cold saltwater would clean out the sand but burn raw flesh. The Corpsman who was assigned to our class was worthless. I never went to him for anything. He would always get the duty vehicle stuck in the sand, and we would have to help un-fuck it. So, I had to figure out some way to bandage my hands. I needed to do it in a gray man way that didn't draw attention to myself.

THINGS LEARNED GOING THROUGH TRAINING

Strip Your Boots

In training, you get issued gear that you will need for training. One of these items is a sweet pair of Bates Lites boots. These are different than the pair you receive in boot camp. They are pretty comfortable out of the box but aren't suitable for training…yet. You will have to doctor these bad boys. You want the boot to be flexible, like a pair of running shoes. The way to achieve this is by removing parts. First, remove the insole. In the heel section of the boot, the first modification occurs. A thick, stiff piece of cardboard wraps around the back of the foot. This needs to be removed as this causes rubbing to the Achilles area of the foot, which forms blisters. You may still get blisters, but it's still a good idea. I used a heat gun and a pair of pliers to do this. Stick the heat gun into the boot to warm up the glue. The boot is held together with industrial adhesive. This is a fire hazard!

After warming the glue, I would use the pliers to pull the cardboard out. This is not a quick process. To do one boot would take me over an hour and a half—next, the toe. Heat the inside of the boot, and I would begin pulling the cardboard. Lastly, the shank is a piece of metal that runs the length of the boot. Some guys removed the shank, but I did not. Once these modifications were made, you had a fresh pair of ready boots to hit the surf with.

Don't do this to your inspection set. Just keep those shined. One thing to note is the sole of the boot is very soft. If you last longer than the first week, you will notice that the heel will wear out quickly. The outside of my heels were shot pretty quickly. There is a lady down the street from training. I won't tell you where; you have to find her yourself. She does resole of the boots.

Another thing to make the boots more comfortable and overall better is soaking them in salt water and wearing them. Luckily, this part happens every time you run on the beach. I kept and put the original insole back after I was done. Some of the guys replace it with an after-market pair. Looking back, I think I would have paid a cash visit to a Podiatrist or a foot products store and gotten custom-made insoles.

Gear Issue

I was issued gear for training when I reported to the Prep school and S.W.C.C. training. This included receiving blouses, trousers, socks, covers, and underwear. Years later, I still wear the same underwear and socks. Other gear consisted of a dive knife, fins, booties, a wetsuit, a UDT vest, etc. We got a checklist and a sea bag when we went through the line to get our gear. As we passed the bins, we would grab items. Always try to get the brand-new shit. The Navy tends to recycle gear used by other candidates before you. The equipment is abused in training. Ripped, torn, broken, missing pieces, rusted, and other damages. Plus, it has someone's name stenciled on it. I would ensure I got one set of uniform items perfect for inspection. By the way, inspections are just another opportunity for a beatdown session. Make sure everything fits or works. We got opportunities for gear exchange if things were F.U.B.R. Make sure you go over your gear as soon as you return to the barracks. Set aside the items that must be exchanged for the next supply run.

Petroleum Jelly

Knives and saltwater do not mix. Being exposed to the water, our dive knives would begin to rust. We would put petroleum jelly on the knife to prevent this from happening when we swam. We would place a glob of jelly behind the ear. After the instructor inspected our knives, we put a jelly layer on the blade before putting the knife in the sheath. The jelly would protect the edge from rust as it does not wash off easily. Applying petroleum jelly saves you from having to deal with the rust later.

Save Your Piss

The water in San Diego is cold, Dam Cold. This meant wetsuits and swim fins. Even with wetsuits, you will be freezing. I would hold my piss until we entered the water. Once We entered the water, ah, the sweet, warm release. We did this to make use of every advantage. Remember, this is not just training but torture to make you quit. At least in my mind, it made me feel warmer. Remember, the training is hell. This trick has been passed down from one class to another for years. Make use of every advantage, or you will not make it. If you're the type of guy that worries about a bit of piss on your skin to survive, then the program might not be for you.

Super Glue Treatment

Remember how I talked about tearing the calluses out of my hands? This is the gray man solution I figured out. At lunchtime, I called my father one day and asked if super glue was safe to put into wounds. He told me it was used for stitches, so it should be safe enough. I didn't have much time because we were about to load up and start the next half of the day. I quickly hung up, dug into my "bud/s box, " a tool bag, retrieved the super glue, and filled the wounds. This first trial didn't work that well. These dried fillings didn't adhere to the wound and fell out with rough evolutions. I tried filling the cavities again but used my shirt to dry the wounds. After wiping out the blood, I would fill the hole and smear the glue on the skin around the wound. With a few minor tweaks, I found a solution. It wasn't perfect or completely comfortable, but it worked. I found that every night, I would need to remove the fillings. The wounds would be goopy the following day if I didn't. I wasn't going to quit. That was not an option. I just had to find a way to keep going.

Food

Going through training, you burn a lot of calories. Until you get to Coronado, you are not served a lot of calories. While in boot camp, we were fed three meals a day. The portions were not training-size portions. They gave us a "fourth" meal each night before bed. This consisted of an apple or banana and what we called a "yoga mom bar," special k bars. It doesn't sound like a fourth meal, does it?

When you go to the galley, go through the line and get whatever they give you. There is a salad bar. This is the part of the galley that isn't portion-controlled. Load up on the tuna fish, pure protein. We would then empty the pan in no time. The galley servers knew we ate the tuna fish, so they would have a pan ready to replace the first one. I would load my plate with tuna and cheese. In addition to eating all of the tuna fish, we would tactfully acquire the peanut butter packets off the table. Smuggling these packets back to our ranks was gold. They made easy snacks or bargaining chips.

For breakfast, the salad bar served cereal, fruit, and yogurt. The yogurt was plain vanilla, and I remember it was pretty good. I would grab a bowl filled with yogurt and granola. I would fill another bowl with Krave cereal. The reason why I got the cereal was not really for the calories. I got it because it was a morale booster to eat chocolate.

Snacks are a must while training. Like I said, you will burn so many calories daily as your job is to work out all day. Every day while in prep school, we were given snack bags. These brown paper sacks were filled with mini Gatorades, raisins, nuts, granola bars, beef jerky, power drink mix, and fresh fruit. They told us that snack bags were part of a research project, so we got to try different things as they added them to the daily rations. Boot camp would greatly appreciate these sacks as the fourth meal.

One of our guys, a former P.J., loved peanut butter cups. They were the perfect snack for the bus ride from one place to another. My go-to was Reese's pieces. I would also get extra sleeves of honey-roasted peanuts. I was never a fan of raisins, so I would find someone to trade with. You want to choose snacks that are going to give you energy. A little bit of sugar does a couple of things. I found that it provides a boost in energy and an increase in morale. Sometimes when things just suck, my 5-meter target was the fact that my bag of Reese's pieces was waiting for me.

You will eat plenty when you get out of prep and on to Coronado. In my opinion, this was the best food in the Navy. It works because the plate is passed from server to server. You only say what you don't want. If you don't say anything, you get everything on the line. There is a self-serve salad and dessert bar. If they still have the butterscotch bars, eat one for me. They were another 5-meter target.

While in Coronado, I would carb load. A few times a week, I would order a medium pizza. We were not allowed to go off base unless the instructors cleared us, which was rare. I could order delivery and pick it up at the gate. I would order either a buffalo or bar-b-que chicken pizza. On the way to the gate, I would swing by the store to buy a large bottle of chocolate milk, a bag of Reese's pieces, a bottle of Pedialyte, and an oatmeal pie.

Hydrate

As you train, you sweat... a lot. Even though this sounds obvious, people don't realize how much they sweat. I had an instructor who would tell us to hydrate during pool evolutions. We didn't think to drink so much water because we thought we weren't sweating in the pool. One day, the instructor told us that even though we were in the pool, we were still sweating and losing water.

When you urinate and sweat, you lose water and electrolytes. I would buy a bottle of Pedialyte, drink half of the bottle straight before bed, and drink the remaining half in the morning. At 5 bucks a bottle, the electrolyte solution wasn't cheap, but I was more than willing to spend the money. I would do this to stay hydrated and have the electrolytes to get through the next day.

Make Them Laugh

If they are laughing, they can't beat you. Okay… they will still beat you, but at least everyone laughs. In training, I learned you need a bit of a sick sense of humor. Even after being S.W.C.C., I realized you must have some type of humor in the military. There will be times when instructors will have some sort of talent show. They will have someone sing, maybe even do a little dance. We were on the pool deck one day in the lean and rest. I guess the instructors heard that one of the students could. So, they told him to sing a song. This guy starts singing Bohemian Rhapsody. The rest of us start singing back while still lean and rest. The instructors also want jokes.

The key to telling jokes, we found, was the darker and sicker, the better. I give you a few jokes. We had this guy the instructors picked on the whole time we were there. He was one tough S.O.B. We were yet again being beaten at the end of the training day. I remember we were all on our backs with heels off the deck 6 inches. And the instructors call out this guy's name and tell him to stand up. What are the instructors telling this guy that he would make him a deal. They would end the beating if this guy could tell them a joke that made them laugh so hard.

He briefly thought about his joke and said, "Instructor, I have a joke." "What's the difference between a Ferrari and a garage full of dead babies?". The instructor replied, "I don't know, what's the difference?" this guy said, "Instructor, I do not have a Ferrari". The entire room erupted in laughter. The instructor then said something like, "I'm convinced that you might actually have a garage full of dead babies". Now, you would have to have known the student to appreciate the whole joke, and I'm not going to go into details out of respect, but you get the idea.

My swim buddy came up with this one joke on the instructor. Let's call the instructor, Smith. He would ask, "What are the four levels of female orgasm?"

Then he would say, "Well, you got the positive orgasm," and he would moan loudly.

"You got the negative orgasm," and he would moan in an unsatisfactory tone.

"You got the normal orgasm," and he would moan in a normal tone.

"Finally, you got the fake orgasm" "Oh, instructor Smith".

As any comedian would probably tell you, know your audience. We would make some dark and raunchy jokes. Nothing seems to be off limits with each other and the instructors. However, we had one instructor who we were told was very religious and did not tell any religious jokes while he was in the space. I will note that I was in the pipeline before the female component was allowed.

I still remember being on the O-course, and during a "mentoring session," one instructor brought up a rumor that the Navy was thinking about adding females to future training classes. You may have to tone down the jokes so as not to upset the female students.

Be Excited To Be There

When you're in the thick of the suck, it can drain your motivation and morale. The days are long. You wake up early and go to bed late. During the training day, you're shuffling from evolution to evolution. Getting the shit kicked out of you with evolutions and constantly reminded that you should just ring out. Though it is sometimes hard to do, be excited that you are there. I remember one day, we were on a run in BUD/S Prep, and we had to run past the building where the BUD/S instructors were. Usually, when we would run past the building, our class leads would want us to be silent, where only our footsteps were the only sound made. One of the guys shouted out, "CLASS THREE ONE EIGHT". Immediately, the entire class shouted back, "HOOYAH THREE ONE EIGHT". The same guy then shouted, "CLASS NINE ZERO". Again, the class shouted back, "HOOYAH NINE ZERO". The class leads were not thrilled with shouting out the class numbers as we passed by the instructor's building.

They assumed that this would have some type of blowback on the class for being disruptive and not practicing being silent operators. Later that day, when we met up with the instructors, I remember when the lead instructor told us that he heard us shouting as we passed by and that he appreciated the pride that we were showing. He also told us that the instructors feed off the class's motivation, and hearing the callouts motivated them.

The lesson learned was always to seem motivated. The training is long, hard, tiring, and stressful. Sounding off loud and proud increases the morale of the class and the instructors. Another thing I recommend is to keep each motivated. I remember one day, we were in a 2-hour beatdown after a long day at Prep school. We were told to get on our backs with the heels raised 6 inches off the deck and then on our stomach in the lean and rest position. My morale was draining back and forth, a series of push-ups and flutter kicks. I remember looking over at my buddy in the next boat crew; he had a big grin. He asked me, "Are we having fun?" I replied, "HOOYAH!". That reminder that we are feeling the same pain and his goofy grin brought me back into the right mindset. Now, I wasn't thinking about… you know, but I was thinking this sucks. My buddy gave me the morale boost I needed in that moment.

I Should have Said NO!

On March 15, 2016, I was dropped from S.W.C.C. class 90. That morning, I sat on the phone with my father as I cried. That morning also served as a painful lesson I have never forgotten. There were 4 of us that were sent to a performance board. I don't remember what the other guys had failed on. For me, it was the O-course and a swim. I had trouble with the Dirty Name and the rope swings. On the weekends, instructors were out on the O-course to help students with obstacles they were struggling with.

The first weekend, one of the instructors (I still remember his name) helped get the balance logs down. I was there every weekend working on issues and had them all down when I got sent to the board. Standing before the Preliminary board, I plead to the instructors to keep and recycle me to the next class. The following day, I was called to the L.T.'s office. I was told to sign this paper. When I was asked why, he told me I was being dropped. I asked, "Aren't I supposed to go before another board?" He said, "Usually, but I just decided because it would take much to get you caught up in holding."

Right then, I should have no! I should have refused to sign that fucking paper. See, what I learned later on in my military career is protocol. We have protocols for a reason. Just like we have instructions. Protocols are go-by during a process. I was supposed to go before two Performance Review boards. I only went to before one. The protocol is two.

I signed because I had only been in the military for a handful of months. In boot camp, they drill in you that when a superior instructs you to do something, you do it. Not doing so is an Article of failure to obey an order. Knowing what I learned after that day, I should have said no. What was he going to do? Send me to Captain Mast. When I got there, I would tell the Captain that he didn't follow protocol. If I said no, there's a chance that I would still be there. He would have made my life hell, but so what, training sucks anyway. You have to learn to embrace the SUCK.

PEOPLE ARE GOING TO QUIT

Going through training, many people will quit. People will quit right in front of you. People will quit before an evolution, and people will quit after one. Your best friend in training will probably quit. One of the toughest things to do is keep training as you watch the instructors escort them away. As selfish as it may seem on the surface, I would look out and say I am still here. The training is a bitch. It's wet, sandy, cold, painful, and miserable. I would sum up in one word: barbaric. Men even attempt because they are different from most. Some may say they are crazy. Those people are right. You have to be crazy to sign up for torture. Remember, some people die during training.

When you are training, you must block out everything. Nothing in this world matters during the training—your wife, mom, dad, sister, brother, girlfriend, kids, dog, etc. You will worry about them as any human would. You will be curious about what they are doing at any moment. The thing is, those thoughts can quickly turn into feeling like you are missing out on something. You are not back at home able to help the wife with the kids, or what if something happens with a parent and you don't hear about it? I would remind myself when these feelings creep in that everyone is okay and fine.

We were on the O-course one day, and the rain fell hard. The droplets were huge and felt like hail when they hit you. The instructors decided to move us into the classroom. In the classroom, one of the instructors asked the students if they had children to stand up. The instructor asked who has more than one child. Some students sat down. More than two? More students sat down. Eventually, one student was still standing, and the instructor asked how many kids he had. I believe the student replied that he had five kids.

Why do guys quit? There are multiple reasons. One guy in my pre-BUD/s class quit because he didn't want to be away from his family and was missing home. Another guy quit because his wife called him and told him that she was pregnant with their first child. Some guys dip their toe in the training, realizing it wasn't for them.

If you have a significant other and you're looking at entering the pipeline, I suggest taking a hard look at your relationship. The pipeline is demanding. I knew one rackmate who got the "dear John" letter during boot camp. He tore her pictures up and probably flushed them.

I will give a few tips: before you start the pipeline, spend loads of time doing all kinds of stuff with her. Make lots of memories for her and any kids you may have. The memories will be helpful for you later when you are in enduring the suck.

DROPPED FROM TRAINING. NOW WHAT?

Let's face it: most guys don't make it through training. The Navy Special Warfare program is, in my opinion, one of the best recruitment tools. Young guys see a television commercial or Navy Seal movie, and all want to be Seals. They rush down to the recruiting office and begin the process. So, what happens when you quit, or you get dropped for some other reason?

After you stop crying about losing your dream job, you return your gear, talk to a chaplain (in my opinion, it is a waste of time), join a working party, and wait to pick a new rate/job. Once you choose a new rate, you wait until they send you to that schoolhouse. I heard that if you went to the chaplain and told him you had failed to adapt, it could be your ticket out of the Navy.

The question is, can you get another contract? If your paperwork states that you are allowed to try again, sure. Just know it will be much more challenging, as I later learned. First, you have to wait a certain amount of time before applying. Second, commands are not going to be helpful. In my experience and those of others I have talked to, command career counselors are unhelpful and mainly unwilling to help. If you want to return, be ready to do a lot of legwork. The competition also gets tougher. You must be blowing PSTs out of the water and submitting top-notch scores.

BUD/s BOX

The following is the list of tools that you will need during training. Nowadays, you can order all these items online and have them shipped. During prep school, I went to Home Depot because they offered a military discount.

1/16 Punch

9/16 Combo wrench

Torch lighter

Brass wire brush

Pliers

Box cutter

Scissors

Sharpening tools (sharpening stone, spend a little extra and get a good one and learn how to use it properly)

Sandpaper (Grit size 400, 600, 800, and 1000)

Duct tape (black)

Electrical (black)

White athletic tape

Packing tape

White-out pen

Super Glue (how many to buy? Yes)

Heat gun (again, buy quality)

Scribe

Dremel tool

3 in 1 oil

WD-40

Never Dull

Naval Jelly

Small ball-peen hammer

Like I said, I bought all the stuff at the local home improvement store in Great "Mistakes" Lakes. All in all, it cost a couple hundred bucks with a military discount. I bought a tool bag to put all this gear in. I recommend purchasing a small hard plastic toolbox or small bucket with a gamma-seal lid to store your fresh new hardware. Make sure you get the one you can screw on and off. The tool bags are cheap Chinese pieces of shit and dry rot easily. Remember, take care of your gear, and it will take care of you.

Other pieces of gear I would recommend getting are dry bags. Again, you can order them online or pick them up at Dick's or R.E.I. Some guys had them and would put their wet gear in them after a swim so they didn't get other stuff wet.

Another piece of gear that I highly recommend is a boot dryer. A boot dryer is a hairdryer for your boot, and it's worth every penny. Your boots are practically soaking wet from when you lace up in the morning till you take them off at the end of the day. The dryer will dry out your boots while you sleep.

I recommend getting the waterproof memo books. They are more expensive than the regular ones, but worth the money. You will carry it with you all the time, whether you are wet or dry.

STOLEN GEAR

Sad as it is to say, people will steal your shit. This has happened to me as well as happened to others. One day, one of the guys stole a rachet wrench off my desk (F.Y.I. buy a few rachet wrenches once you get out to Coronado; there's a hardware store right up the street from the base.) as I worked on my gear. I must turn away for a second as I didn't see him do it. Once I knew it was missing, I asked, and no one had it. Then I found it in the guy's tool bag. No one had the brand that I had. This guy had stolen various things from other people as well.

I suggest buying paint or getting some color spray can plastic and paint your tools yellow or pink or whatever. This is what I thought about doing after it happened to me: painting all my tools pink. Another thing you could do is engrave all of your tools by scratching identifiers such as names or symbols. If you went with the bucket for your tool's idea, make a few modifications. Screw the lid on and cut a hole in the top of the cover near the edge. Cut another hole in the side of the bucket. Once you have done this, run the length of the chain through both holes and connect the ends with a lock.

Last Word

I hope this guide helps you along your journey, becoming the less than 1% of the population to be an operator, let alone even have the balls to attempt. The journey is long and hard. Never give up, never ring out. The last piece of advice is to skip serious girlfriend relationships or get the girl pregnant. I watch guys quit because of it. Good Luck!

OFFICIAL PST LOG

Here is a template to get started with logging your PST scores.

DATE:		DATE:		DATE:	
SWIM 500 YARDS		SWIM 500 YARDS		SWIM 500 YARDS	
PUSH UP		PUSH UP		PUSH UP	
SIT UP		SIT UP		SIT UP	
PULL UP		PULL UP		PULL UP	
RUN 1.5 MILES		RUN 1.5 MILES		RUN 1.5 MILES	
DATE:		DATE:		DATE:	
SWIM 500 YARDS		SWIM 500 YARDS		SWIM 500 YARDS	
PUSH UP		PUSH UP		PUSH UP	
SIT UP		SIT UP		SIT UP	
PULL UP		PULL UP		PULL UP	
RUN 1.5 MILES		RUN 1.5 MILES		RUN 1.5 MILES	

DATE:		DATE:		DATE:	
SWIM 500 YARDS		SWIM 500 YARDS		SWIM 500 YARDS	
PUSH UP		PUSH UP		PUSH UP	
SIT UP		SIT UP		SIT UP	
PULL UP		PULL UP		PULL UP	
RUN 1.5 MILES		RUN 1.5 MILES		RUN 1.5 MILES	

DATE:		DATE:		DATE:	
SWIM 500 YARDS		SWIM 500 YARDS		SWIM 500 YARDS	
PUSH UP		PUSH UP		PUSH UP	
SIT UP		SIT UP		SIT UP	
PULL UP		PULL UP		PULL UP	
RUN 1.5 MILES		RUN 1.5 MILES		RUN 1.5 MILES	

RANDY HUGHES

DATE:		DATE:		DATE:	
SWIM 500 YARDS		SWIM 500 YARDS		SWIM 500 YARDS	
PUSH UP		PUSH UP		PUSH UP	
SIT UP		SIT UP		SIT UP	
PULL UP		PULL UP		PULL UP	
RUN 1.5 MILES		RUN 1.5 MILES		RUN 1.5 MILES	
DATE:		DATE:		DATE:	
SWIM 500 YARDS		SWIM 500 YARDS		SWIM 500 YARDS	
PUSH UP		PUSH UP		PUSH UP	
SIT UP		SIT UP		SIT UP	
PULL UP		PULL UP		PULL UP	
RUN 1.5 MILES		RUN 1.5 MILES		RUN 1.5 MILES	
DATE:		DATE:		DATE:	
SWIM 500 YARDS		SWIM 500 YARDS		SWIM 500 YARDS	
PUSH UP		PUSH UP		PUSH UP	
SIT UP		SIT UP		SIT UP	
PULL UP		PULL UP		PULL UP	
RUN 1.5 MILES		RUN 1.5 MILES		RUN 1.5 MILES	
DATE:		DATE:		DATE:	
SWIM 500 YARDS		SWIM 500 YARDS		SWIM 500 YARDS	
PUSH UP		PUSH UP		PUSH UP	
SIT UP		SIT UP		SIT UP	
PULL UP		PULL UP		PULL UP	
RUN 1.5 MILES		RUN 1.5 MILES		RUN 1.5 MILES	

MOCK PST

This is for you to record unofficial practice PST scores. Treat it like the real deal by sticking to strict time rest limits. 10 minutes rest after swim, 2 minutes after push-ups, 2 minutes after sit-ups, and 10 minutes after pull-ups. Good integrity practice.

DATE:		DATE:		DATE:	
SWIM 500 YARDS		SWIM 500 YARDS		SWIM 500 YARDS	
PUSH UP		PUSH UP		PUSH UP	
SIT UP		SIT UP		SIT UP	
PULL UP		PULL UP		PULL UP	
RUN 1.5 MILES		RUN 1.5 MILES		RUN 1.5 MILES	
DATE:		DATE:		DATE:	
SWIM 500 YARDS		SWIM 500 YARDS		SWIM 500 YARDS	
PUSH UP		PUSH UP		PUSH UP	
SIT UP		SIT UP		SIT UP	
PULL UP		PULL UP		PULL UP	
RUN 1.5 MILES		RUN 1.5 MILES		RUN 1.5 MILES	
DATE:		DATE:		DATE:	
SWIM 500 YARDS		SWIM 500 YARDS		SWIM 500 YARDS	
PUSH UP		PUSH UP		PUSH UP	
SIT UP		SIT UP		SIT UP	
PULL UP		PULL UP		PULL UP	
RUN 1.5 MILES		RUN 1.5 MILES		RUN 1.5 MILES	
DATE:		DATE:		DATE:	
SWIM 500 YARDS		SWIM 500 YARDS		SWIM 500 YARDS	
PUSH UP		PUSH UP		PUSH UP	
SIT UP		SIT UP		SIT UP	
PULL UP		PULL UP		PULL UP	
RUN 1.5 MILES		RUN 1.5 MILES		RUN 1.5 MILES	

RANDY HUGHES

DATE:		DATE:		DATE:	
SWIM 500 YARDS		SWIM 500 YARDS		SWIM 500 YARDS	
PUSH UP		PUSH UP		PUSH UP	
SIT UP		SIT UP		SIT UP	
PULL UP		PULL UP		PULL UP	
RUN 1.5 MILES		RUN 1.5 MILES		RUN 1.5 MILES	
DATE:		DATE:		DATE:	
SWIM 500 YARDS		SWIM 500 YARDS		SWIM 500 YARDS	
PUSH UP		PUSH UP		PUSH UP	
SIT UP		SIT UP		SIT UP	
PULL UP		PULL UP		PULL UP	
RUN 1.5 MILES		RUN 1.5 MILES		RUN 1.5 MILES	
DATE:		DATE:		DATE:	
SWIM 500 YARDS		SWIM 500 YARDS		SWIM 500 YARDS	
PUSH UP		PUSH UP		PUSH UP	
SIT UP		SIT UP		SIT UP	
PULL UP		PULL UP		PULL UP	
RUN 1.5 MILES		RUN 1.5 MILES		RUN 1.5 MILES	
DATE:		DATE:		DATE:	
SWIM 500 YARDS		SWIM 500 YARDS		SWIM 500 YARDS	
PUSH UP		PUSH UP		PUSH UP	
SIT UP		SIT UP		SIT UP	
PULL UP		PULL UP		PULL UP	
RUN 1.5 MILES		RUN 1.5 MILES		RUN 1.5 MILES	
DATE:		DATE:		DATE:	
SWIM 500 YARDS		SWIM 500 YARDS		SWIM 500 YARDS	
PUSH UP		PUSH UP		PUSH UP	
SIT UP		SIT UP		SIT UP	
PULL UP		PULL UP		PULL UP	
RUN 1.5 MILES		RUN 1.5 MILES		RUN 1.5 MILES	
DATE:		DATE:		DATE:	
SWIM 500 YARDS		SWIM 500 YARDS		SWIM 500 YARDS	
PUSH UP		PUSH UP		PUSH UP	
SIT UP		SIT UP		SIT UP	
PULL UP		PULL UP		PULL UP	
RUN 1.5 MILES		RUN 1.5 MILES		RUN 1.5 MILES	

MEAL TRACKER

Eat right to train right. Here is a food intake tracker.

DATE	DATE	DATE	DATE	DATE
BREAKFAST	BREAKFAST	BREAKFAST	BREAKFAST	BREAKFAST
LUNCH	LUNCH	LUNCH	LUNCH	LUNCH
DINNER	DINNER	DINNER	DINNER	DINNER
SNACKS	SNACKS	SNACKS	SNACKS	SNACKS

DATE	DATE	DATE	DATE	DATE
BREAKFAST	**BREAKFAST**	**BREAKFAST**	**BREAKFAST**	**BREAKFAST**
LUNCH	**LUNCH**	**LUNCH**	**LUNCH**	**LUNCH**
DINNER	**DINNER**	**DINNER**	**DINNER**	**DINNER**
SNACKS	**SNACKS**	**SNACKS**	**SNACKS**	**SNACKS**

THE TRAINIG GUIDE I WISH I HAD

DATE	DATE	DATE	DATE	DATE
BREAKFAST	BREAKFAST	BREAKFAST	BREAKFAST	BREAKFAST
LUNCH	LUNCH	LUNCH	LUNCH	LUNCH
DINNER	DINNER	DINNER	DINNER	DINNER
SNACKS	SNACKS	SNACKS	SNACKS	SNACKS

DATE	DATE	DATE	DATE	DATE
BREAKFAST	BREAKFAST	BREAKFAST	BREAKFAST	BREAKFAST
LUNCH	LUNCH	LUNCH	LUNCH	LUNCH
DINNER	DINNER	DINNER	DINNER	DINNER
SNACKS	SNACKS	SNACKS	SNACKS	SNACKS

DON'T QUIT!

Made in the USA
Coppell, TX
12 July 2024

34564039R00036